WALTZING WITH ALZHEIMER'S

# WALTZING WITH ALZHEIMER'S

## Caring When
## Your Partner
## Is Out Of Step

DANIEL TYLER

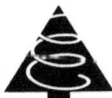

SPRING CEDARS

Cover art by Lauren Zurcher
Cover and book design by Spring Cedars

ISBN 978-1-963117-10-3 (paperback)
ISBN 978-1-963117-11-0 (ebook)

Published by Spring Cedars
Denver, Colorado
www.springcedars.com

*For Dan and Patty Henshaw.*
*Your support made all the difference.*

It would be foolish of me to suggest that my exposure to dementia mirrors that of the millions of people worldwide who suffer with the disease or act as caregivers. Each experience is just too individual. However, I was a caregiver for my partner over the last half of our twenty-year relationship and during that time, I learned that we were part of a unique community, dealing with stresses and burdens that are difficult for outsiders to comprehend. While individual challenges may be different among us, we have much in common. Because I was a caregiver, I feel inspired to tell my story complete with lessons learned, mistakes made, problems solved and unsolved, and the emotional battles I survived. My hope is that anyone beginning to deal with dementia will benefit from my tale. Dementia is a rough ride for anyone, and its course is maddeningly irregular, painfully cruel, and often of a duration that challenges our patience, our health, and our finances.

To better understand the depth and power of this tragedy as it affected me, I want to set the stage by describing the life Betty and I enjoyed before she was diagnosed with Alzheimer's disease (AD). It's the only way I know to effectively present the devastation and the loss that descend on both the sufferer and the caregiver. We do all we can to assist a loved one with AD, but we eventually need professional assistance and there just isn't enough to go around. Betty and I witnessed the best and the worst forms of care. Our experiences made an indelible impression on me. They serve as the principal reason why I conclude with an appeal to the Alzheimer's Association to invest in developing a professional caregiver training program.

Betty and I met when I was living in Steamboat Springs, Colorado, and she was living in Cincinnati, Ohio. I was divorced and looking for a chance at a mutually congenial partnership. After graduating from the University of Nebraska, Betty trained as a special education teacher and took a job at an elementary school in Long Beach, California, where she met her husband. After marriage and a few years in Cambridge, Massachusetts, where Ed earned an MD degree from Harvard Medical School, they moved to New York where he conducted cancer research at the University of Rochester. Betty raised their son, Dan, in Rochester and developed a business selling tiled, wrought-iron tables. Unfortunately, her husband developed prostate cancer and died following a radical

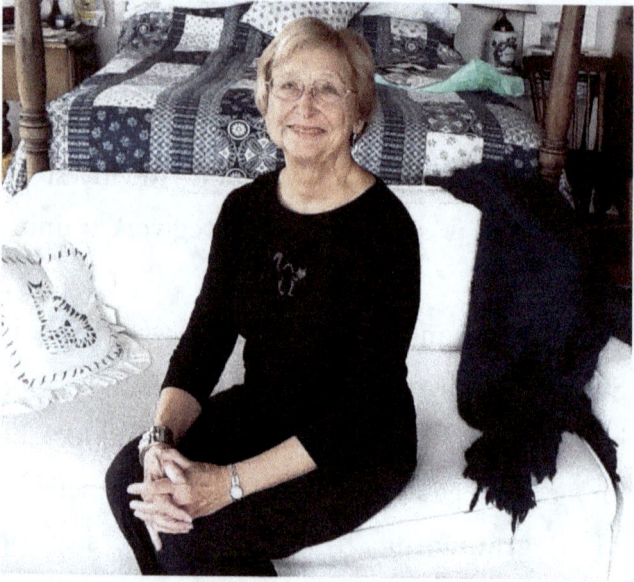

*Betty's Cincinnati apartment, 2003*

treatment. Betty moved to Cincinnati to care for her aging mother-in-law.

I, too, graduated from Harvard. Hoping to attract a lady with similar educational and cultural instincts, I composed an ad for the personals section of the Harvard Alumni Bulletin. When the magazine appeared with my ad, Betty had already buried her mother-in-law and was emerging from almost a decade of grieving for her husband.

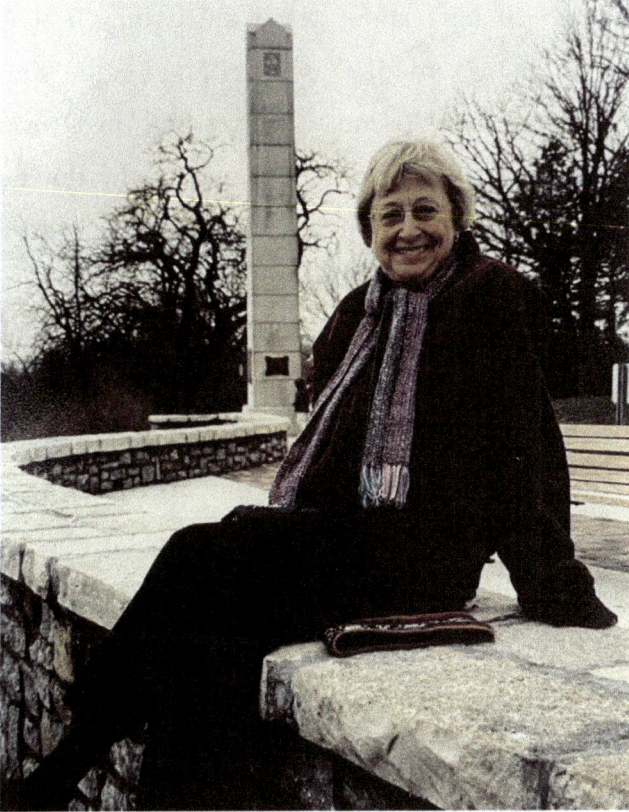

*At the Ohio River historical plaque, 2003*

At $5 a letter, my ad was short: "Retired university professor (history), sixtyish, looking for kind, optimistic, upbeat, generous woman to share outdoor interests . . . in Colorado Rockies. rockydan@aol.com."

"I don't know why I am writing," Betty replied by email, "as I clipped out your 'personal' for a friend who lives both in Denver and SF. As I reread it, I thought why don't I write, as I think of myself as 'optimistic, upbeat and generous with outdoor interests?'"

Obviously we didn't know it at the time, but this was the beginning of a twenty-year relationship. Both of us were brand new to courting of any sort and only because Betty continued to receive and read her late husband's Bulletin did she see my ad. For my part, placing the ad was a long shot. My residence was in Colorado, and most of the action in the Bulletin took place between men and women in the East.

Communication between us continued via email and was good from the start. We got the big subjects out of the way early on: sex, religion, and politics. We exchanged pictures and after a couple of months, there was enough interest to warrant my making a trip to Cincinnati. Betty was living in a top-floor apartment overlooking the Ohio River. The views were

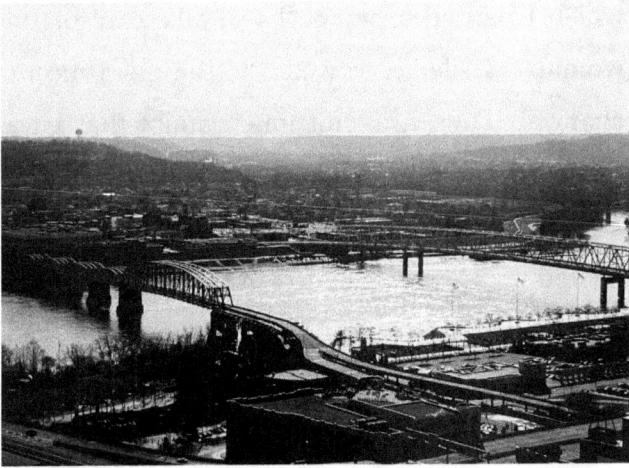

*Ohio River from Betty's apartment*

extraordinary. I found myself developing a warm feeling about her as we toured the city and visited the farm in Shandon, Ohio, half of which she had recently inherited from her late mother-in-law. It was clear that she was comfortable in both the city and the country; she was down to earth and well read. She was scarred from several tragedies and openly emotional about her losses, but she was also tough, resilient, and optimistic. I became increasingly drawn to her. Just prior to my departure, I saw a picture of her late husband which I paused to view. "I will take care of this woman," I silently vowed, "if she gives me the chance." There was not much doubt that I was falling in love and the feelings were mutual.

Soon after returning to Colorado, Betty invited me to visit her in Hawaii. She traveled to Oahu every winter to be with her son, Dr. Dan, who was a radiologist at Kaiser Permanente in Honolulu. Dr. Dan was married with two young children, and he lived in Kailua on the east side of Oahu, a thirty-minute drive from his job. Betty had been renting a house for half a dozen years on Lanikai Beach, about a mile away from her son's home. It was rustic; doors didn't always close, the TV stopped working on occasion, the furniture was old and well used, appliances hummed in concert with each other, and the cockroaches were large, fast, and hungry. But from the back door, the ocean was less than 50 yards away. The waves were small, the water was warm, and the beach was idyllic. Having taught at Punahou School in Honolulu for five years after my discharge from the Air Force, I was

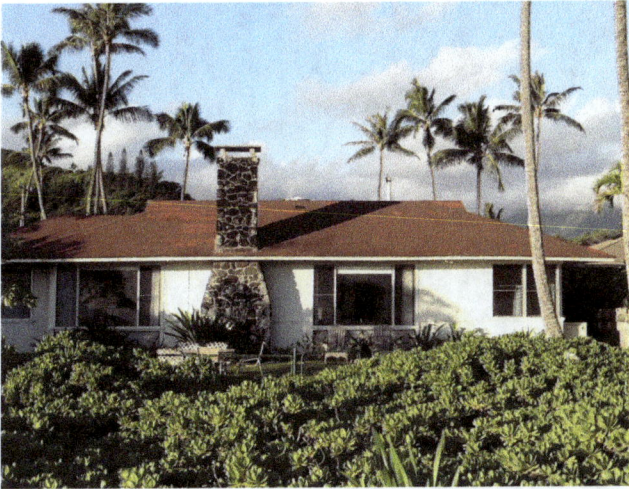

*Lanikai beach house*

quite familiar with the islands, and I did not hesitate to accept Betty's invitation.

My first visit lasted two weeks. Over the next 12 years, we made the Hawaii winter pilgrimage annually, staying for increasing lengths of time. In that tropical setting, there was nothing that had to be done and there was, at the same time, lots to do. We cared for Dr. Dan's children when their parents wanted a mainland break. We golfed together—Betty didn't play but loved to ride with me through the jungle that was The Royal Hawaiian Golf Club. We welcomed

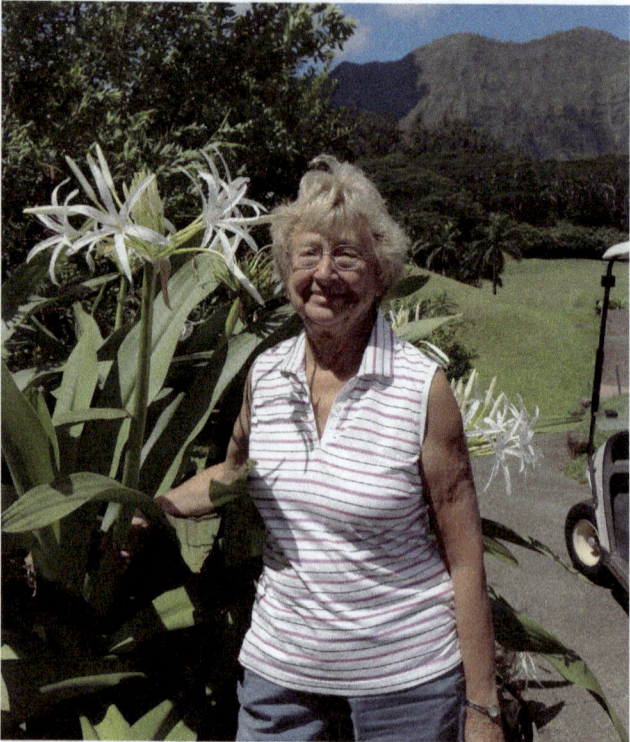

*Hawaii Spider Lily bush at Royal Hawaiian Golf Club*

mainland guests, walked Lanikai Beach at dawn with a cup of coffee, and enjoyed an occasional evening meal at Buzz's Steak House or, on special occasions, at Mariposa, an elegant Neiman Marcus bistro with lanai seating and views of Waikiki Beach. Betty hosted her mainland friends in 2006 for a celebration of her 70th birthday,

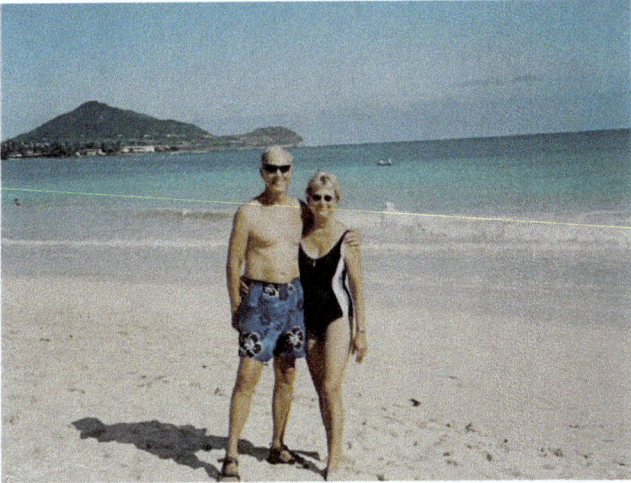

*On Lanikai Beach*

complete with luau and hula dancing. Everything we did in Hawaii was great fun.

When not in Hawaii, we hung out at my place in Steamboat Springs or at Betty's apartment in Cincinnati. The warmer parts of the year were perfect in the Colorado mountains, but our time in Ohio was also filled with enjoyable activities, family, and friends. Traveling back and forth between the two states was easy; we often went alone but always anticipated the pleasure of getting back together after short separations.

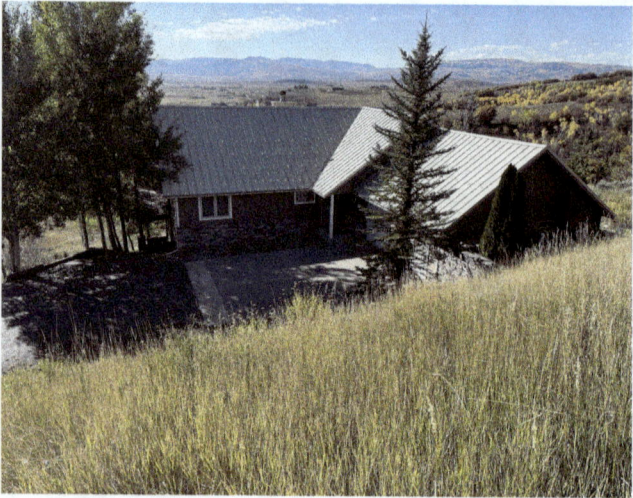

*Steamboat house*

The richness of the first 10 years of our relationship was enhanced by many adventures. Our travels all over the country included visits to Santa Fe, Sedona and Lake Powell, Banff and Lake Louise in Canada, Martha's Vineyard and the site of the 1889 Johnstown flood in Pennsylvania. We took in the Reno Air Races, watched high-performance vehicles at the Bonneville Salt Flats, and paid a visit to the Flight 93 Memorial crash site near Shanksville, Pennsylvania. We attended my 50th Harvard reunion, joined a week-long tour following

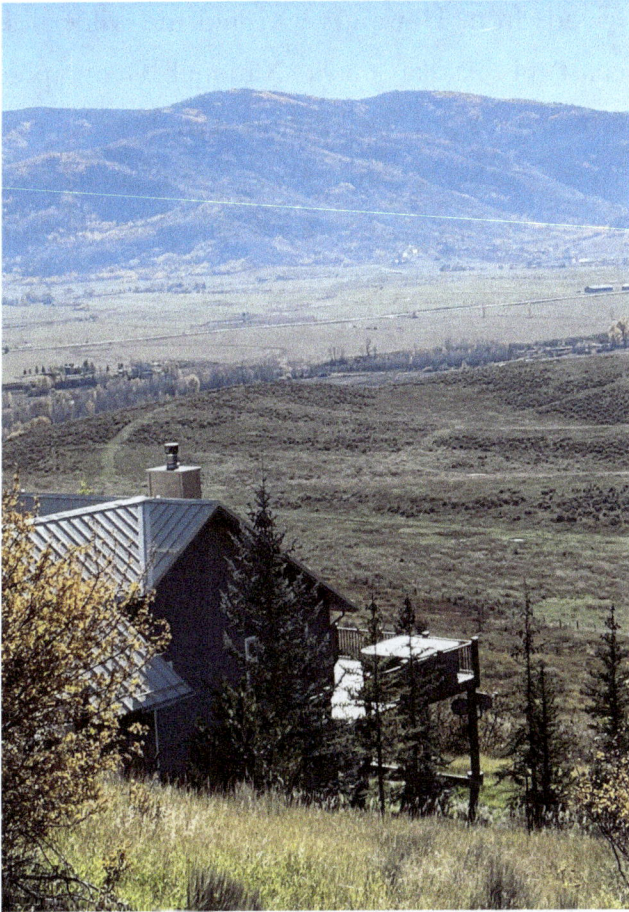

*Steamboat house with deck and hot tub*

Benjamin Franklin in Paris, took in a concert at Carnegie Hall, camped out in a Nebraska hut to watch Sandhill Cranes, and visited Butchart Gardens in Victoria, British Columbia. With friends from Hawaii, we visited the wilderness coast of Alaska on a National Geographic cruise, took in Frank Lloyd Wright's Taliesin West in Scottsdale, Arizona, attended the Kentucky Derby, and joined forces with my son to drive his Triumph TR-3 from Philadelphia to San Rafael, California, with other vintage cars in what had become known as The Great Race. We attended professional baseball games, toured the United States Air Force Museum in Dayton, Ohio, shared the "joys" of doing research for three books (*Love in an Envelope*, *Mum*, and *Cowboy in the Boardroom*), searched for humpback whales from the back seat of a glider off Kaena Point in Hawaii, and reveled in the incredible highs of a mutually supportive relationship. Although my two marriages had their share of good times, I had not known until then the serendipitous joy of such an effortless relationship. You could say that I was about as content as one can get in a relationship when the crash occurred.

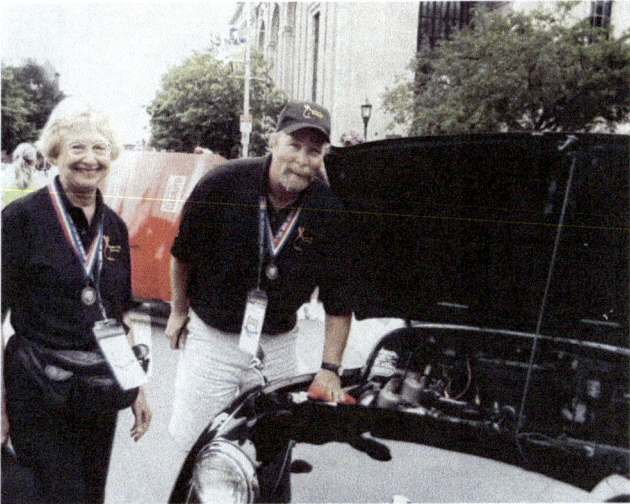

*Betty and Nick Tyler, The Great Race*

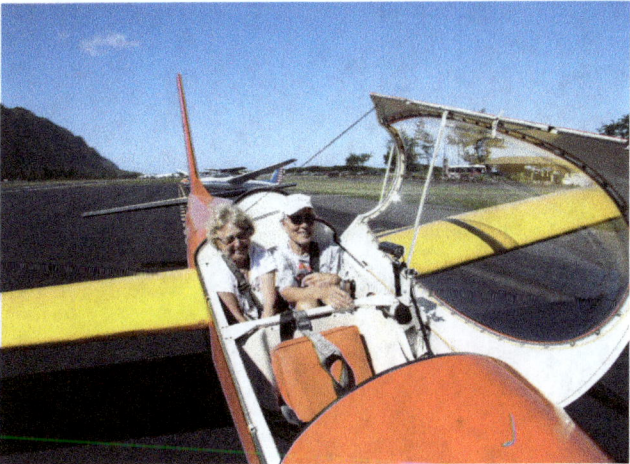

*Glider flying*

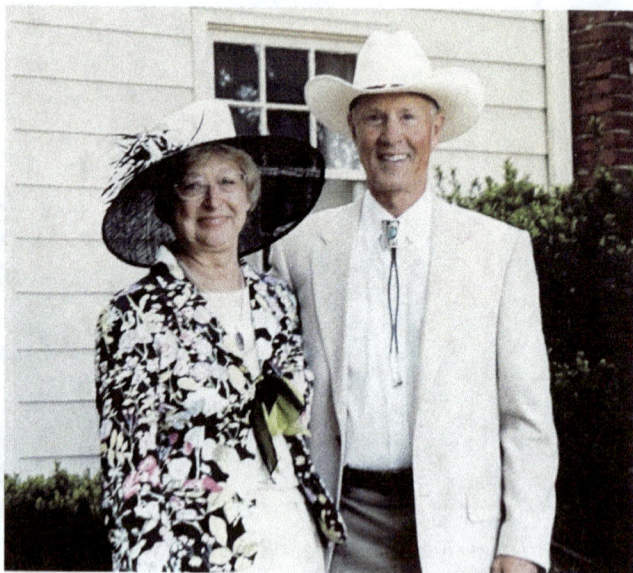

*Dan and Betty at Kentucky Derby*

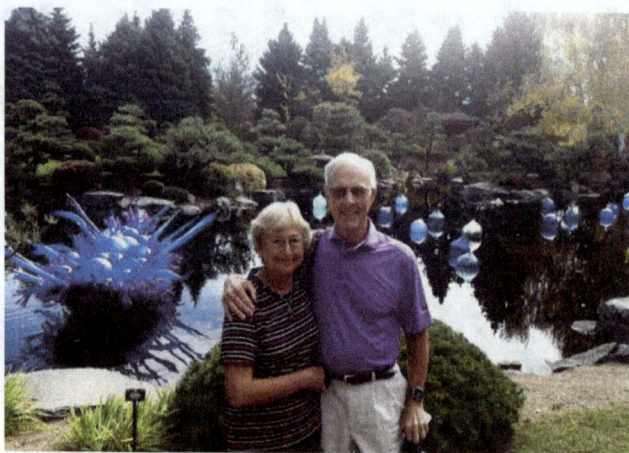

*Denver Botanic Gardens*

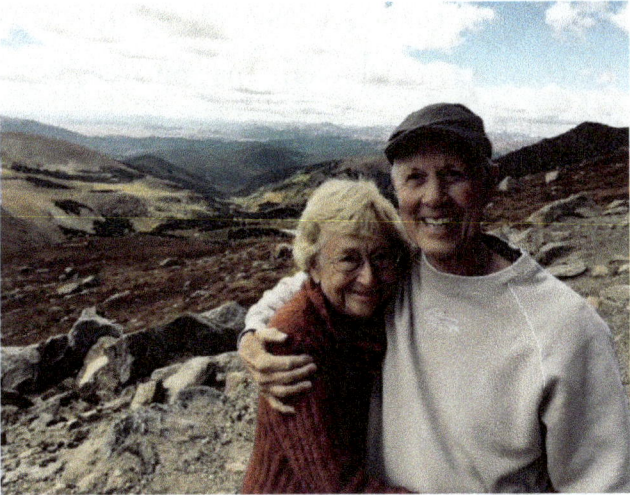

*Climbing Mt. Evans*

The emotional shock of what happened next can be attributed to my denial of the old proverb that nothing lasts forever and that all good things must come to an end. I will always recall with sadness how it felt to realize that something unwelcome had entered our relationship, subverting the good chemistry and causing me to feel concerned and a tad frightened.

In 2012, Betty announced that she wanted to sell her half of the Shandon farm to her brother-in-law and move her principal residence to Colorado. She wanted to buy an apartment in Denver. In some ways, I understood her reasoning. Her brother-in-law owned the other half of the farm, and he wanted to spend more time there with his daughters and their children. He lived in North Carolina and found it awkward to have to coordinate with Betty every time he wanted to gather his family. He wasn't a farmer in any sense of the word, but it was his family's property and for him the experience was going home.

For almost 10 years, Betty and I had traveled between Colorado and Ohio without any fuss over the brief periods that we were apart. We both had spent the solo time feathering our respective nests and re-charging batteries in anticipation of another visit; another adventure. I was sorry to see this pattern end, but it was clear that Betty was determined to make the move, and I went along with it, trusting that our lives would continue to be seamlessly magical. Betty found an apartment on the 36th floor of a relatively new downtown building, across from the Denver Convention Center with views that extended from Longs Peak in the north to Pikes Peak in the south. With floor-to-ceiling glass windows in several rooms, three elevators, a 24-hour concierge, parking for two cars, and an open-air area for barbecuing, hot tubbing, and social gatherings, The Spire presented a new style of living that felt quite exhilarating.

With the purchase complete, we addressed what I thought would be a simple matter of furnishing the apartment. I've never had strong feelings about household furniture; I'm far more dedicated to comfort than fashion. So, I was happy to be guided by whatever Betty wanted, expecting to act as an occasional arbiter when she had trouble making a decision. But that was not how the furnishing process unfolded. We found a great furniture store and a savvy sales person who had plenty of ideas and what appeared to be a pretty good understanding of how Betty and I lived. But when it came to

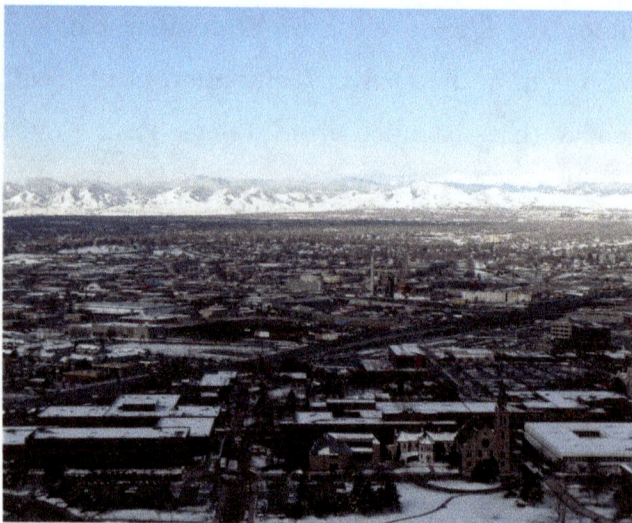

*Spire view from living room*

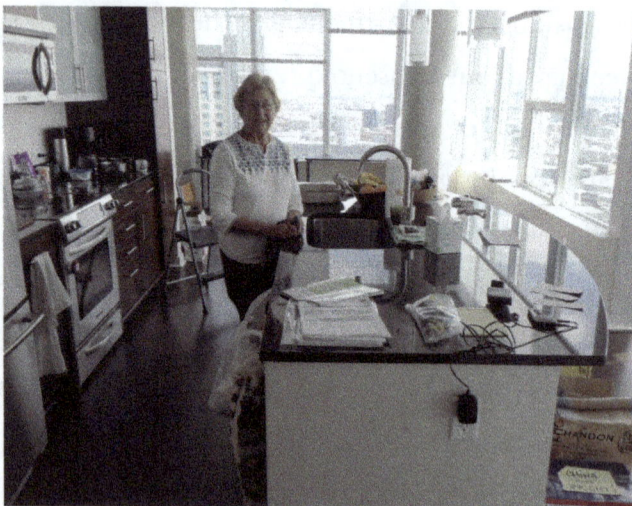

*Spire kitchen*

actually making a decision on specific pieces, Betty was flummoxed. She wanted me to decide on everything. This was so unlike her. I asked myself, "What's going on here?" She left a lovely apartment and a farm which she knew well. She loved to entertain at the farm, and she customized the property by bringing over an 1850s log cabin that she tore apart and rebuilt as an exact replica of a pioneer home. Her mark on that farm was unique. It was where she was most in her element. But she preferred to leave all that behind and come to Colorado where she had only a few casual acquaintances, no family, just me. And then she bailed out of any responsibility for furniture decisions, perfectly content to have me do it all. What was going on?

I really twisted and turned trying to answer that question. I called Dr. Dan to ask him if he had noticed anything the last time we were in Hawaii. Neither one of us had any idea what was happening, although Betty's hearing was getting worse. Dr. Dan surmised that perhaps she just needed new hearing aids.

It wasn't for almost a year after noticing other small changes in Betty's behavior that I realized that we were probably dealing with something more than hearing loss. She had begun to lose confidence in herself. She was fearful of making decisions on her own. Even at restaurants, she tended to wait until I ordered so she could request the same thing, knowing that it would be an acceptable choice. Her move out of Ohio, I finally concluded, had to do with her need to lean on me for support and assistance. She never expressed what she was feeling. She might have had some awareness of her changing behaviors, but she never shared her concerns. Neither one of us knew at the time that these insecurities were the beginning signs of some form of dementia, but I was quite aware that the balance and easygoing flow in our relationship had changed. I had to be very careful about comments that might sound critical to her. The relaxed, intuitive comfort of our relationship had taken a body blow. Little did we know how much more punishment was awaiting us down the road. I had just become a caregiver, and I really had no idea what I was doing.

For a year or so, I didn't feel like we were fighting off anything too serious. Dr. Dan didn't seem too concerned either, so I tried not to worry. Ninety percent of the time, Betty and I continued as we had in the past. But there were times when I felt like I was walking on eggshells, and I could see that Betty was beginning to need lots of reassurance. I had to revise the way we interacted, leading gently while trying not to show frustration when the comfortable patterns of our relationship shifted. Because we were both ignorant of the reality of her condition, the elephant in the room remained relatively unnoticed for several years, making our relationship at times feel somewhat awkward. I remember clearly the first time I commented on her forgetting something she had always known. She jumped on me for being critical. "My husband was never critical of me," she announced. I became abruptly aware of how important my words and my body language were going to be moving forward, and I felt challenged to be everything Betty expected me to be. I just didn't know what we were dealing with.

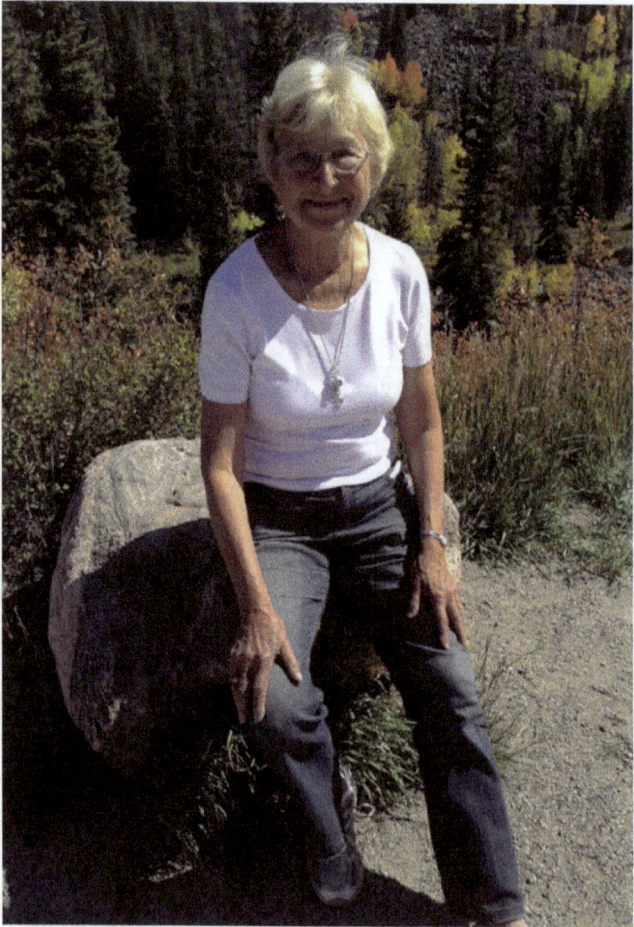

*Blue River Canyon*

During our Hawaii sojourn in the winter of 2013–2014, I tried to persuade Dr. Dan that Betty should see a specialist. He was reluctant to make an appointment, still believing that Betty's issues had more to do with hearing loss, variable sleep patterns, and the onset of frequent urinary tract infections. In the spring, when Betty joined the hiking group with which she had been touring the UK annually for almost 20 years, I warned one of her Cincinnati friends that they might want to keep an eye on her. The "American Ladies," as they called themselves, were good friends, and they knew each other very well. The anomalies in Betty's behavior, I surmised, would be noticeable quickly, and the group needed to be prepared.

It wasn't long before my fears were confirmed. Betty had an old Blackberry cell phone. She was relentless about keeping it on her person in a charged condition, hoping to remain in contact with me. Not long into the trip, she texted me that she was fine but ready to come home. Shortly thereafter, her companions wrote me with observations that hit hard. Betty had ignored packing instructions and only had light, summer clothes; she was often confused about the day's hike; she wasn't bathing regularly, and her short-term memory was unreliable. She was still good company and seemed to be enjoying herself, but they were worried about her.

"Betty requires daily care," they wrote me. "She cannot live alone. She is compulsively addicted to her Blackberry, is reluctant to let it out of her sight, and gets confused about how to work it. She shouldn't be handling her own medicines, has no concept of time, and is quite stubborn. This is a marathon, and you have had the longest run. It's time to pass off the baton to her son."

In a certain sense, I felt some relief. Betty's behavioral condition was not a figment of my imagination. Caring for her had become part of the daily planning process for a group of women who had known her longer than I had. But handing her off to Dr. Dan was out of the question. He was still working long hours at Kaiser, and I still hadn't persuaded him that his mom might have some form of dementia. I now understand and empathize with his reluctance to make this determination. He was already aware that his atrial fibrillation had been passed on genetically by Betty, and the possibility of dementia in his future was not a welcome thought. But we needed an evaluation by a neurologist, and he agreed to make an appointment with Dr. Michiko Bruno in Honolulu.

When the three of us visited Dr. Bruno in 2015, she asked Betty questions and ordered an MRI. When we returned to the clinic for an assessment of Dr. Bruno's findings, we were told that Betty's frontal lobes appeared to be in retreat and although she could not be absolutely certain, Dr. Bruno concluded that Betty was probably in the beginning stages of Alzheimer's disease.

I remember walking out of the clinic feeling stunned. I did not know much about AD, but the diagnosis made sense given what I had witnessed in the previous three years. When we got to the car and closed the doors, I turned to

Betty and told her that we were at a watershed moment and that it would be necessary for her to use her brain as much as possible in the days ahead. I told her we were in this together, that I would be by her side at all times, and that we would find a way to make the best of a nasty situation. She stared at me like a deer caught in the headlights, didn't say a word, and showed no signs of emotion at all. I'm sure she was confident that I could fix whatever was happening to her, but I felt devastated. I knew that our future was going to be a lot different than what I had experienced for the past 10 years.

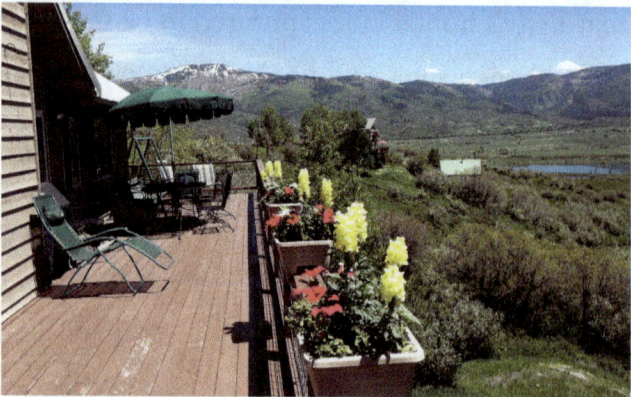

*Betty's flowers in Steamboat*

The remainder of 2015 underscored how our relationship was evolving. Betty's restlessness at night impacted my sleep, especially in Denver where street noise was pronounced. I had some grumpy days. But she continued her creative cultivation of flowers in Denver and in Steamboat and thoroughly enjoyed the time we spent in her apartment, where we attended shows at the Denver Center for the Performing Arts, a few baseball games, and made the most of Denver's culinary highlights. In general, life was good, but my caregiver role was becoming more complex and weighty. I started overseeing Betty's financial affairs to make sure that bills were paid and accounts were not overdrawn. I made all her appointments with hairdressers, doctors, and an attorney who drew up a new will and a power of attorney that divided responsibility for Betty's care between me and Dr. Dan. Although Betty and I weren't married, I was in effect her legal partner. She had assets to manage and was often visited by representatives from the trust companies and banks that handled her affairs. It was my duty to explain what was going on with Betty and because I was uncertain how her AD would develop, I often found myself in an uncomfortable role, lacking confidence in the advice I gave. But that's the nature of caregiving; a lot of guesswork! I had become the go-to person and while Betty was delighted with my role as her informal advisor, advocate, and spokesperson, I became increasingly nervous about all the duties I was taking over and how our relationship would play out as time wore on. From lover, best friend, and confidante, I felt myself becoming Betty's supervisor. I was determined to do my best, as I had vowed to her late husband, but I began to wonder how long I could last without help. And when I did take time for myself, I felt guilty.

In the winter of 2015–2016, Betty traveled to Hawaii with an Omaha cousin and her husband. The plan was for the three of them to stay in Betty's Lanikai Beach rental for a couple of weeks while I attended to chores in Steamboat. Everyone knew about Betty's tendency to develop UTIs in Hawaii, but this time the infection arrived quickly accompanied by severe pain. When I arrived, Betty was feeling miserable and her cousins couldn't wait for me to take over. Welcome to paradise!

The next day, we were at the urologist's office. Because of Betty's UTI history, the doctor took aggressive steps to examine her thoroughly. I'm not sure what he did exactly, but he probed and poked and scraped looking for suspicious bacteria. Finding nothing, he sent us home without much more than an offer to see her again if symptoms persisted. And they did. In fact, they got worse. We returned to the doctor the next day. By the time we headed home, Betty was shaking uncontrollably. She had developed a high fever and was very uncomfortable. I called Dr. Dan. He came to the house and saw that we had an emergency on our hands. Betty was showing signs of sepsis. Dr. Dan rushed her to the nearby Adventist Health Hospital where she received heavy doses of antibiotics. Her condition was serious enough to require around-the-clock observation.

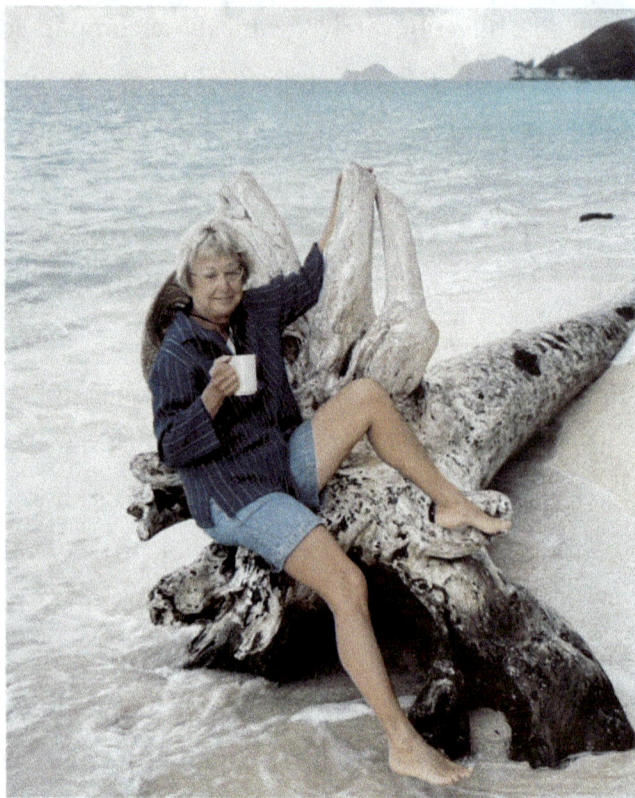

*Morning coffee*

She recovered but returned to the rental
house fatigued, confused, and weak. Every day
that passed, she got a little better, but I had to
stay with her most of the time. Dr. Dan kindly
hired caregivers from a company that employed
wives of Marines stationed at nearby Marine

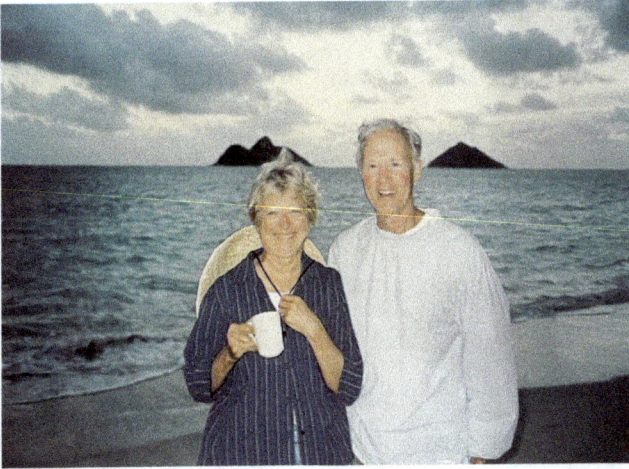

*Betty and me in Hawaii*

Corps Base Hawaii. They were nice ladies but totally ignorant of the idiosyncrasies of dementia. They came to babysit, and Betty soon grew tired of their presence in her home. She felt that her private space was being invaded by people she didn't know and because different caregivers showed up each day, she refused to interact with any of them. She was occasionally quite blunt, even suggesting they go home. The caregivers made it possible for me to enjoy some time on my own, knowing that at least Betty was safe, but I didn't have much fun. Betty just wasn't happy, so our first experience with hired caregivers was a bust. The ladies weren't professional, and Betty's negativity provided me with a first glimpse of how AD accentuates a person's determination to maintain some control of daily life, making decisions, feeling useful, and wanting to be needed.

The power of these emotions became increasingly evident a few weeks later. I had invited my children to join us in Kailua for spring break, and they were due to arrive in a few weeks. My initial inclination was to cancel the invitation, but they really wanted to come and my doctor daughter-in-law assured me that they would be easy guests. When the two adults and two children arrived, Betty's demeanor changed completely. All of a sudden she perked up. Most of her life she had been a great hostess, so when my family arrived, those instincts kicked in. She was still confused occasionally, but the presence of guests for 10 days did more to brighten her spirits than anything else I could have done. AD attacks and weakens the logical functioning of the brain, but the senses actually grow stronger. Anyone who is in a caregiving role needs to understand this: a caregiver's looks and facial expressions say more than words, while touch and feelings need to be nurtured to establish trust.

When the family departed, I sat down with Dr. Dan and his wife, Patty, to discuss our future. I can't say enough about my good fortune of having really fine people to deal with under very trying circumstances. For so many families, figuring out the best way to deal with an aging relative with AD is fraught with baggage from the past, jealousies, financial concerns, geography, and many other issues. Solutions are hard to come by, because a life is at stake and not everyone recognizes the need to help and the importance of working together. Little differences of opinion, life's ups and downs, can destroy family harmony when AD appears.

Conversations for us were hard, but they were honest and sensitively delivered. We needed to agree on where Betty would live as the AD worsened. Dr. Dan was her only child, but he was reticent about having her move to Hawaii. I knew that Patty was also concerned about Betty staying in the Islands, because her own mother was in her nineties. Although she was still physically strong and intellectually competent, a time would come fairly soon when she might need her daughter's assistance. The thought of having two older ladies to care for simultaneously was not especially palatable. Dr. Dan still worked long hours. There was no way he would be able to help care for his mom during the 5–6 days he was at the radiology department in the hospital.

I was of two minds about what to do. A part of me wanted to assume all the caregiving, not just because of the vow I made to Betty's late husband, but because I knew that Betty wanted me to be in charge. Moving to Hawaii in her later years was not an option she had ever mentioned during the dozen years we had been a couple. She had told me on various occasions before the AD arrived that if anything happened to me, she would want to return to her roots in Nebraska. On the other hand, I could feel the beginnings of stress associated with the level of caregiving I was already doing. It seemed to me that if Betty was ever to return to her son, now was the time, because travel would be more difficult the older she got. And these were my thoughts five years before COVID struck.

Ultimately, I asked Dr. Dan to come to Colorado for a few days to see if together we might be able to interest his mom in an assisted living facility. He agreed. With Betty in tow, we made appointments to tour several CCRCs (Continuing Care Retirement Community) in the Denver area.

They all appeared to be nice places, but Betty was unimpressed. She was beginning to sense that she was about to be abandoned and to some extent, she was right. I was beginning to feel that I couldn't do an adequate job of caregiving alone without giving up many aspects of my own life, including a strong sense of responsibility to my own children and grandchildren. This was selfish on my part, but I wanted to do the work necessary to patch up earlier years of neglect when I was busy trying to make a success of my teaching career. And I had obstacles to surmount as a result of earlier missteps.

When Betty's Omaha cousin informed us that there was a really nice facility nearby and that she would be willing to act as Betty's advocate if she came to live there, Dr. Dan and I jumped at the prospect of a solution to the stalemate we had encountered in Denver. The three of us flew to Omaha and drove directly to the facility. Dr. Dan asked me to wait in the lobby while he and Betty toured the complex. They ended up in a conference room to hammer out the details of Betty's move, but she was having none of it. If she were moved to Omaha, Betty made clear, she would just stop eating. Dr. Dan was on the verge of tears. He came to the lobby to get me, hoping that I could change his mom's attitude, but when I entered the room, I could tell she was very angry. There was nothing I could do. We were at a standoff. Betty felt that she had been ganged up on by her own family, and she was furious. I couldn't blame her.

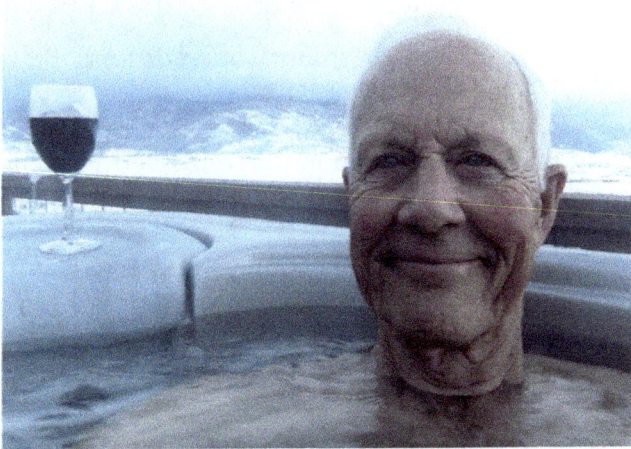

*Hot tub*

Following a tense meal at a lovely restaurant, we flew home. Betty gradually relaxed when we settled into my house in Steamboat. That's where she wanted to be. But I was a mess, and Dr. Dan wasn't far behind. I had no idea what to do next, nor did he.

Sitting in my hot tub with a cup of coffee the next morning, I watched the sun rise after a restless night. It seemed to me that someone had to step up to the plate, so when Dr. Dan came out on the deck to join me, I told him that I had decided to sell my house and move with his mom into Casey's Pond, Steamboat's local CCRC. We would stay there together, I offered, until Betty needed the next level of care or required the kind of medical attention that only Denver could provide. Coming to this decision caused me a lot of anguish. I loved the only home I had ever built, and I dreaded the thought of trading the views, the peace and quiet, and the neighbors for residence in a facility dedicated to the care of seniors with age-related mental issues. I also knew that if Betty and I were to remain together, I would need caregiving assistance, and that would be a lot harder to come by were we to stay in my house in the country; especially during winter months. But I also felt that I was doing the right thing. Betty would be one hundred percent happy anywhere with me, and all the anger that had risen up in Omaha would be forgotten. Needless to say, Dr. Dan was also pleased and relieved. Looking back, I'd say I hit a home run.

My house sold quickly. Casey's Pond offered us a unit on the third floor which had a view of the ski mountain, a generously sized

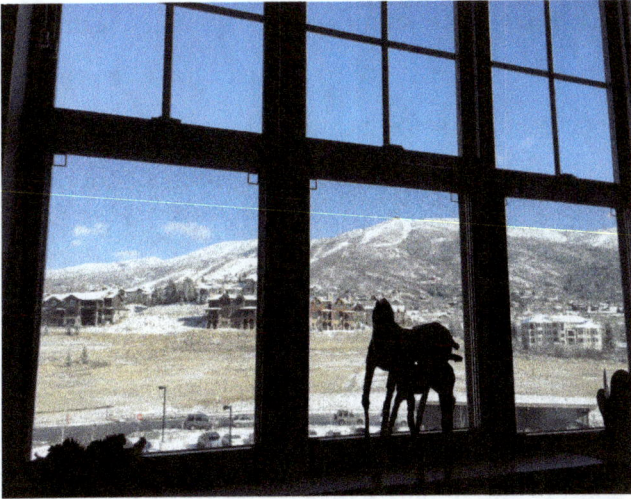

*View from Casey's Pond*

living room, bedroom, small kitchen, and a windowless study. It was quite nice. Betty loved it. We furnished it with some of our possessions from my house. Everything else went into storage nearby. As the winter closed in, we settled into a new routine. I skied every other day and found companion caregivers for Betty when I was on the mountain. She was quite content with this routine. We ate our meals together in the main dining room and made a few friends. But most residents were sedentary, and some were experiencing dementia. I felt awkward and out of place, so when Dr. Dan arrived to take Betty to Hawaii for Christmas, I decided to look for a different arrangement.

My first choice was Betty's condo in Denver. I am not all that comfortable in a city; too many wonderful years on my dad's ranch on the Western Slope had inculcated in me a love of the outdoors where I feel freer and more relaxed. But we had spent short periods of time at the condo, and I had learned to enjoy some of its conveniences as well as its unique location for entertainment and dining. The City Park Golf Course, Botanical Gardens, and Coors Field (baseball) were close by as well as many other cultural facilities. While Betty was in Hawaii, I checked us out of Casey's Pond and moved our things to Denver. By the time Betty returned from Hawaii, I had added items to the condo, making it homier and more familiar to her. Betty's artwork was on the walls, and the two parking spaces in the building would make it easy for family and friends to visit.

Betty was delighted and so was Dr. Dan.

Patty found a licensed social worker online who advertised caregiving in private homes. She had a stable of ladies who worked for her and when we met, I was impressed by her business acumen. She appeared smart, interested in helping us, and determined to select caregivers who would relate well to Betty. Dr. Dan and I agreed to work with her. We set up a schedule that provided Betty with companions 4–5 days a week. Betty and I still ventured out together for meals and an occasional excursion, but for the first couple of months at the condo, I was able to spend more time with my grandchildren while Betty was being cared for. I was really happy to have the freedom to develop a good connection with my family. Living in Steamboat was everything I had hoped for, but while Betty and I lived there and in Cincinnati, I had neglected my family.

I even played a little golf on the days when Betty was being cared for. On one outing at an executive course called The Links, I noticed a "For Sale by Owner" sign on a house which backed up to the 16th fairway. I called the

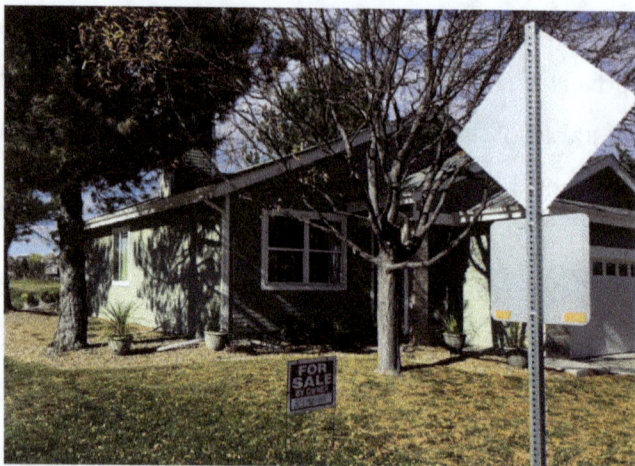

*House on The Links Golf Course*

owner and made an appointment to see it the next day. It occurred to me that, perhaps, Betty and I might live there if we tired of the city. I showed her the house, and I know she would have moved there had I insisted, but I could tell that her heart wasn't in it. Knowing that at some point Betty would have to enter a CCRC, I decided to buy the house anyway. It needed some remodeling, so I spent the next few months overseeing some upgrades while making use of the garage to store my stuff. I was in no rush to move in, but the location close to my children and grandchildren seemed like a good place for my future, even if I wasn't able to occupy it right away.

Every day that I worked on the house, Betty had caregiver companions who took her to eat, grocery shopping, and to various places of interest. These ladies wrote notes to me, summarizing their day with Betty, commenting on her general state of mind and any behavioral idiosyncracies I should be aware of. They did a fine job, and I reciprocated with suggestions of my own regarding Betty's needs. I learned from their notes that Betty was becoming increasingly confused. She was asking a lot of questions about most aspects of her life and was rarely satisfied with a single answer. She had trouble following through on promises to improve bodily hygiene and got her back up when she felt pressured to fulfill expectations. As she had demonstrated in Hawaii, maintaining some control of her life was important. When the ladies appeared to be taking over or passing judgment, she became belligerent. They liked her, however, and the caregiver relationships were generally positive. On occasion they would indicate in their notes that Betty had moments of sadness and depression, that she seemed to be fearful of the dark, and that she was sometimes rude to waiters at restaurants. She desperately wanted to feel productive and useful, so I hired an artist to give her abstract painting lessons once a week. She loved the artwork and raved about the time she spent with Santiago, but he began taking advantage of me, insisting that I pay him in advance. Eventually, he just didn't show up and walked away with a large chunk of my money.

By the fall of 2017, I had decided that it was time to seek out a licensed therapist whose understanding of dementia might allow us to make progress in finding an appropriate CCRC for Betty. I could tell that I was wearing down, and I hoped that someone with geriatric expertise might find ways to persuade Betty to transfer into an independent living facility. To some extent, my plan succeeded. Betty began to talk more about the pros and cons of staying in the condo. She knew that I had taken on considerable responsibility for her care, but in the recesses of her mind she still embraced the idea that any move would have to involve me as well.

Unfortunately, the social worker in charge of Betty's caregivers got wind of our conversations with the therapist. She was already miffed over my opposition to her earlier attempt to move Betty into a CCRC of her own choosing. She never asked my advice, but she persuaded Dr. Dan that his mom would be better off in a small facility neither one of us had ever heard of. Dr. Dan called me to announce a forthcoming move. I was shocked, and I balked, using my POA, explaining to Dr. Dan that I didn't want Betty to be placed in a facility that I hadn't carefully investigated. He felt badly about having agreed to the move, apologizing immediately. I now realize that his willingness to allow his mom to be moved had been a result of knowing that my job was becoming increasingly difficult and that some kind of move in the not-too-distant future was in the cards for all of us. As busy as he was, Dr. Dan was actually trying to ease my burdens, and I thanked him for that. What he didn't know was that when openings occurred, the facility in question rewarded referrals with a significant amount of cash. Losing out on this bonus caused our social worker to become vindictive.

Her response was immediate. All caregivers she had been providing for the previous 10 months were removed. We were left on our own. For a social worker to behave like this is inexcusable, but the lesson learned simply added to others we had experienced regarding the unsettled, unregulated, and sometimes unprofessional world of caregiving. I filed a complaint with the State of Colorado, but it languished in the bureaucracy for two years, eventually resulting in a mild reprimand for the social worker.

Now that Betty seemed more amenable to discussing a move out of the condo, I decided to become more aggressive. I began by looking at Balfour at River Front Park, a new CCRC on the South Platte River that was nearing completion and was situated close to Betty's condo. It appeared to be thoughtfully designed, with nicely appointed apartments, trained medical personnel on staff, and an adjoining memory care facility that would be seamlessly available to residents when their dementia required upgraded care. I took Betty with me when I had appointments at Balfour. She joined me for meals in the dining room, participated in discussions with staff, and walked with me to get a feel of the neighborhood, but her enthusiasm was modest at best. In the deep recesses of that damaged mind, she sensed that something wasn't quite right. Even though I always referred to a potential move as something we would be doing together, she was suspicious; abandonment was her greatest fear. I did my best to overcome her reluctance. I hired an expensive decorator to furnish the apartment, hung pictures on the walls, and placed knick-knacks she would appreciate as an artist, but she could never get past the feeling that once removed from her condo, she would never return and I would leave her. On the day we agreed to move in for a two-week trial, I had our bags packed at the door of the condo, when she sat down and refused to move. We never stayed a day at Balfour, and I ended up donating all the furnishings to my daughter and losing a $15,000 deposit to Balfour.

This was a real low point for me. For being a reasonably intelligent and common sense sort of guy, I felt like a giant failure: my lovely Steamboat house was gone; I was unable to accommodate to life at Casey's Pond; I had caused the loss of caregivers for Betty at the condo; I was unwilling to bring Betty to my golf course home; and I had taken a big financial hit at Balfour. I felt empty, fragile, and frustrated. Working with dementia should not be so difficult, but it was and it is. Over the 10 years I dealt with Betty's dementia, I learned that everyone who is a caregiver has to get used to setbacks. Logic and practicality can be maddeningly absent from the equation. You have to recognize the dominant role of feelings, and you have to approach difficult decisions with a firm understanding that what might work one day may be inappropriate the next. Caregiving, whether by family members or paid companions, is a rollercoaster experience. It's frustrating, and it's exhausting. Perhaps, the most important lesson caregivers need is the importance of flexibility, tolerance, understanding, and respect, all set against the background of an Alice-in-Wonderland environment where up is down and down is up. A modicum of success is possible with AD sufferers, but there must be trust between caregiver and patient. The journey toward trust can be twisty and uneven, but if it can be developed, caregivers can lead. I was just figuring that out.

I decided that it was time to be more decisive and to show Betty that I knew what I was doing. For several months, I had been attending an Alzheimer's support group in order to learn from others with similar experiences.

Some discussions were helpful; others were self-serving and redundant. The best information I received was about a woman who had a reputation for persuading dementia sufferers to leave their homes and enter a CCRC. She was also good at dealing with families and helping them choose the right facility. Most of the good places had waitlists; some were large, some were small, some were owned by investors, some were advertised as non-profit. To the uninitiated, making a choice was like buying tires. Having someone with experience to guide Betty and me through the selection process was just what I needed.

Ginny turned out to be as good as her reputation. She showed up at my home with an attorney who specialized in family law. We sat on my porch while I described Betty's condition, the sharing arrangement I had with her son, and the overall course of Betty's AD we had been witnessing for the previous five years. The two women were emotionally supportive, upbeat, and committed to helping me. We discussed the pros and cons of various CCRCs and agreed to tour a few places they thought might be a fit. We ended up looking at three. The last one, Cherry Hills Assisted Living and Memory Care (CHAL), had been open only a few months. Ginny was experienced enough to know that it usually took a few years to determine the quality of the management team. But she liked the open feeling at CHAL with its many floor to ceiling windows and its location overlooking the lovely DeKoevend Park. We arranged for a tour. In addition to the feeling of newness, CHAL was bright and peaceful. It was spacious and well designed. Access to the park was relatively simple, and Goodson Recreation Center was adjacent to the parking lot. I knew how much Betty liked the outdoors. CHAL felt like it was part of nature, and I sensed that she might enjoy living there, even though the facility was relatively immature and untested.

I contacted Dr. Dan and told him we should move his mom to CHAL as soon as possible. He was supportive. They had an available room close to the front desk with three windows that overlooked the park. I found a company that specialized in one-day moves. They took pride in recreating the feel and physical structure of a client's home—downsized and in miniature—so that everything appeared to be included in the new space: clothes in the closets, pictures on the walls, books on the nightstands, etc. I urged Dr. Dan to come to Colorado as soon as possible so we could move Betty into her new home together. We would also stay with her for a few nights until she became familiar with the routines. He agreed.

After briefing the mover on essential items to be brought over from the condo and showing her the space she would be working with at CHAL, we scheduled a date for the move. Dr. Dan arrived a few days before the transfer so we could have the semblance of a normal visit. On the appointed day, the three of us departed the condo and headed for Rocky Mountain National Park. We left early and took a picnic. Betty was delighted to be having a day

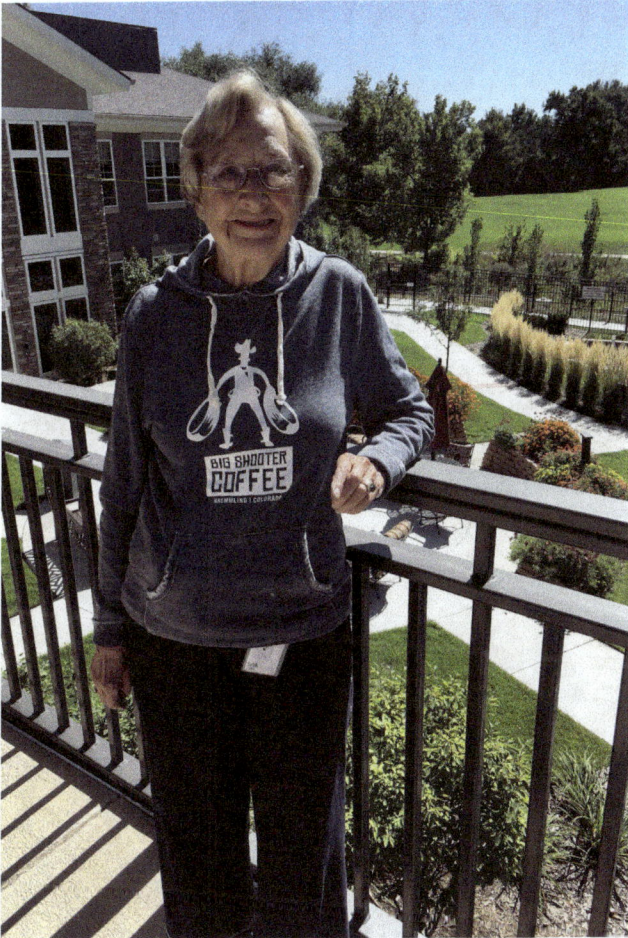

*Betty on CHAL porch overlooking DeKoevend Park*

in the country with her two Dans. It was October, and the leaves on the trees were gorgeous. The drive over the Continental

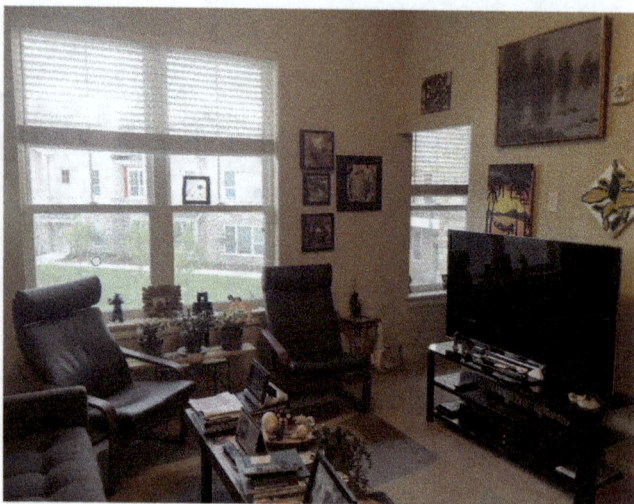

*Betty's living room at CHAL*

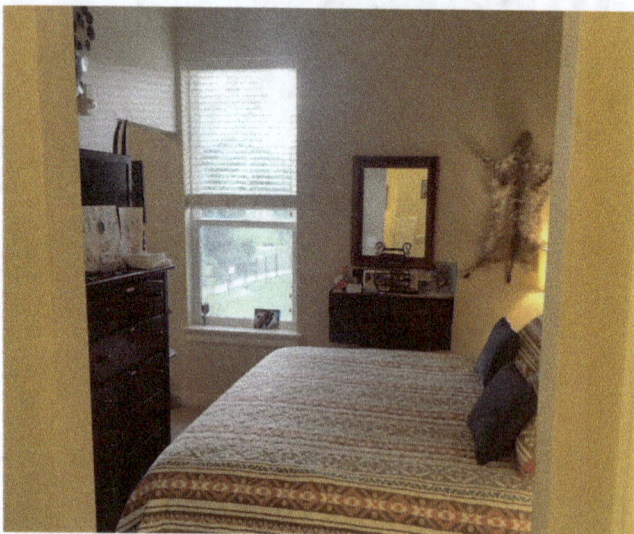

*Betty's bedroom at CHAL*

Divide's Trail Ridge Road provided us with spectacular views, and the elk herds showed up as if by appointment. Along with a cobalt blue sky, a warm sun for our picnic, and no wind, the day was magical. Around 4PM, we started back to Denver, arriving at CHAL about 5:30PM. We said very little to Betty about the future, simply noting that we would all be staying together for a while. Betty said nothing about all her belongings being so carefully arranged in the new space, and she seemed relaxed and happy. We had supper in the dining room and watched TV with Betty before retiring for the night—Dr. Dan on the living room sofa, Betty and I in the same bed she had been sleeping on in her condo.

Looking back, I suspect that Betty knew something had changed in her life. She was aware that she wasn't at her condo, but because Dr. Dan and I avoided any discussions about the past or the future, she was content to follow our lead. The part of her mind that occasionally produced fear and caused negative behaviors was quiescent. She felt secure around us, accompanied by her possessions. The unfamiliar nature of the new location, the strange faces in the building, and an altered routine did not seem to cause unrest. We were all living in the moment, precisely what AD sufferers want and need.

Dr. Dan stayed for a few days then returned to Hawaii. I remained with Betty for more than a week, until the director suggested that I was overstaying my welcome. I told Betty that I had to go away for a few days. By then, she had become somewhat familiar with the new routines: when and where to eat; who would provide her medications; fitness class; art activities, etc. She still retained a tight grip on her Blackberry, but that actually proved helpful. Whenever she needed answers, she could call me. And occasionally, she would just call because she wanted reassurance.

For the first few months, we developed new ways to connect. I started living in my golf course home, about four miles south of CHAL. I made regular visits, joining Betty for a meal,

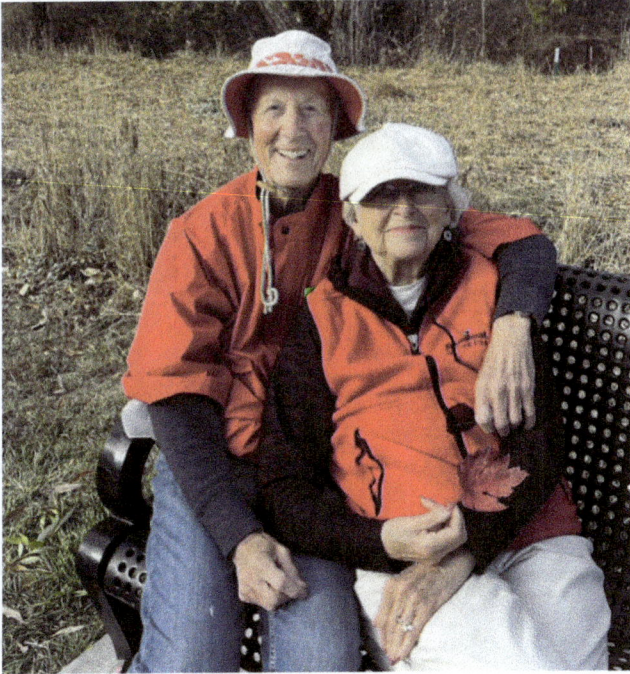

*DeKoevend Park*

taking her for a walk in the park or along the nearby Highline Canal, and accompanying her on occasion when she had an interesting art class. She always wanted me to stay longer, hoping I would bring my grandchildren for meals and spend the night. It was very hard to say goodbye, but I finally learned to respond positively to most of her requests. When I did

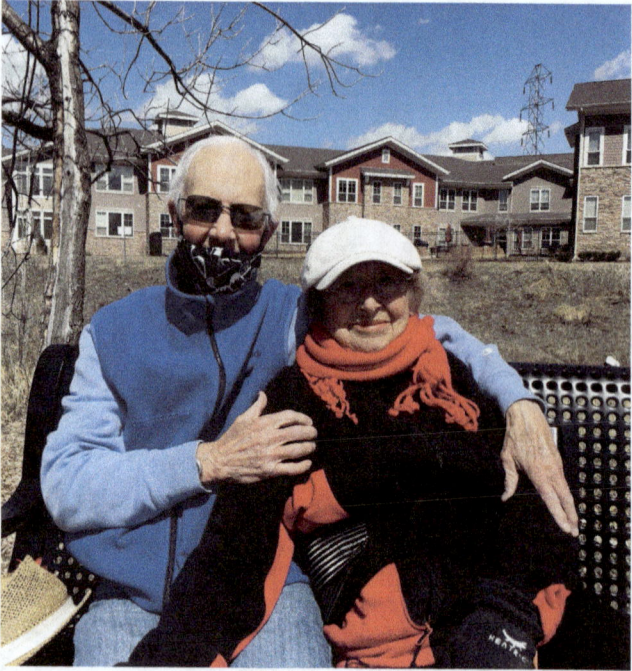

*DeKoevend Park with CHAL in the background*

this—when I was positive about things—she would relax and I could leave. Whatever I had promised would be forgotten in short order. I was lying to her. It hurt to do this. I agonized over the repeated prevarications and drove home angry with myself, beating on the steering wheel, sometimes in tears. I was dealing with loss and even though CHAL was able to provide Betty with security, potential new friends, and some interesting activities, I felt guilty. I was giving up much of my previous caregiving responsibilities to a for-profit facility that was charging an outrageous amount of money for its services. I felt like I was letting down the one I loved, to whose late husband I had made a vow of love and protection. I missed terribly the person I had found 15 years earlier. I was lonely, damn it!

But as the months turned into years— Betty remained at CHAL for four and a half years—I came to realize that I could not have been her only caregiver without doing myself irreparable harm. I was still very much a part of her care, dealing with everything from medical appointments and hairdressers to actively monitoring her treatment at CHAL. She would eat with other residents, but most of her time was spent doing crossword puzzles in a chair adjacent to the facility's main entrance. She liked being close to the comings and goings of providers, visitors, and CHAL personnel. Occasionally, I arrived when she was taking a nap in her favorite chair. I would sneak up behind her and plant a kiss on her neck. She would jump at the unexpected touch. The staff loved it and when she was ready, we would take off on an ice cream run in her car or head out on one of our walks.

At first, we walked about a mile on the Highline Canal. There was a broad path for walkers, runners, bikers, and horses. She loved watching the ducks in the canal, the hawks in the trees, and all the blooming flowers and other greenery. There were benches along the trail where we could sit together. She loved these moments. They were serene and joyful for both of us. I learned to slow down, enjoy just holding hands, and watch the clouds roll by. Betty would sometimes put her head on my shoulder and doze off. When awake, she would frequently express how happy she was, how she couldn't imagine being in a more perfect place. As her back started to bother her, we shortened our walks and spent more time sitting on a bench in DeKoevend Park. We were entertained by all the

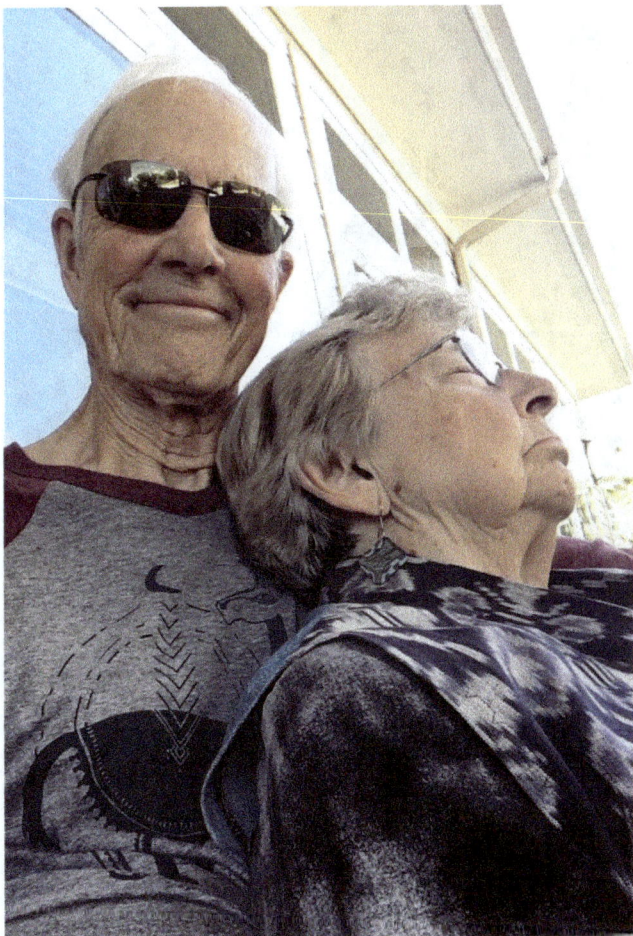

*Betty asleep under CHAL portico*

activities, especially the dog walkers who frequently introduced their pets to us. Betty loved to take naps if the sun was warm and

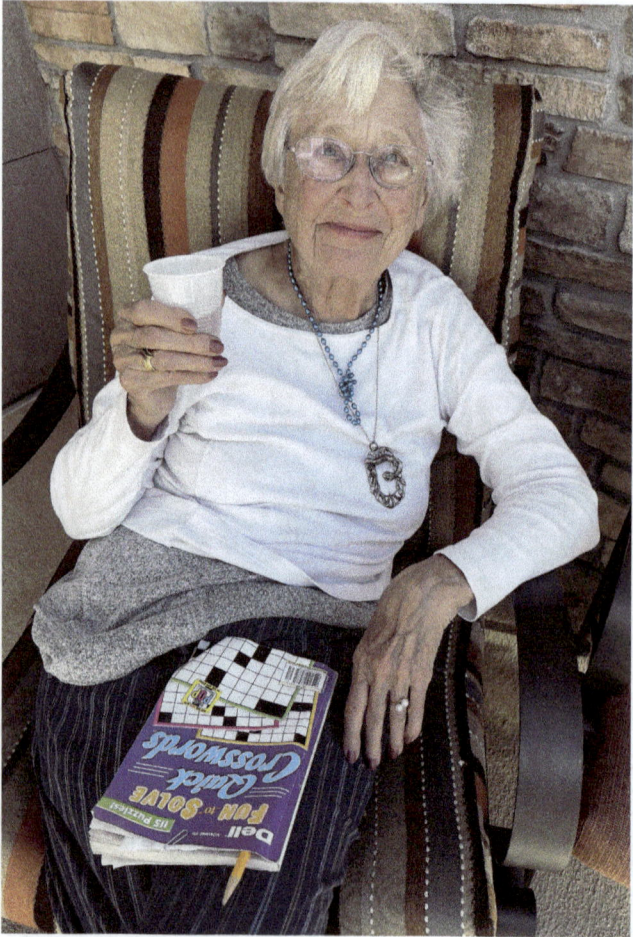

*Betty with her crosswords*

because she leaned on me to get comfortable, I would sometimes have to wake her up due to excruciating pain in some part of my anatomy or

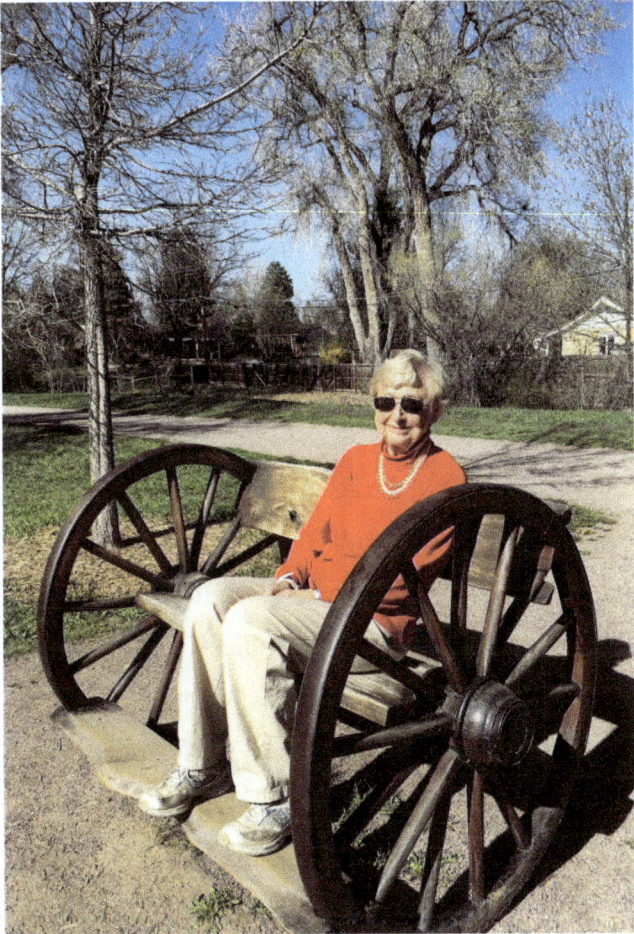

*Highline Canal*

a limb that had gone to sleep and was totally useless. But as her back began to ache more, I struggled to get her outdoors. Returning to the building proved an enormous challenge, and I could always tell when she was hurting badly.

During winter months, we went on short drives, sometimes for ice cream or later in the evening, to see the Christmas lights during the holidays. I took her with me when the Denver Ukulele Orchestra had practices on Sunday nights in Lakewood, but she was so fearful of the dark that I had to end those excursions. Prior to every New Year, I raised money for the CHAL staff as a way to thank underpaid caregivers for their service. We did pretty well, thanks to the generosity of CHAL's families. Betty couldn't help me with the fundraising, but she sat beside me when we doled out cash to all the QMAPs (Qualified Medication Administration Personnel), and she was thrilled by the hugs and occasional tears from those who received the gifts. She was happy to be doing something useful. She felt needed and appreciated.

Occasionally, we sat on the porch overlooking DeKoevend Park. I played the guitar for her or helped her work on sticker puzzle books. Her needs were simple: affection, understanding, encouragement, and touch. I would have been a better caregiver during those years had I known of Owen Darnell's lovely 2013 poem titled "Do Not Ask Me to Remember":

Do not ask me to remember
Don't try to make me understand
Let me rest and know you're with me
Kiss my cheek and hold my hand
I'm confused beyond your concept
I'm sad and sick and lost
All I know is that I need you
To be with me at all cost
Please don't lose your patience with me
Don't scold or curse or cry
I can't help the way I'm acting
I can't be different though I try
Just remember that I need you
That the best of me is gone
Please don't fail to stand beside me
Love me 'til my life is gone

Betty was never mean-spirited or demanding. She always reflected the essence of grace and beauty that had been a hallmark of her life. She was loved by the staff for her gentleness and the one-liners that made them laugh. But she wasn't social; AD had eroded her confidence, and hearing loss exacerbated her preference for isolation. As CHAL's budgets got tighter and fewer employees were forced to deal with a full complement of residents, activities began to decline. I tried to make up for the shortages by increasing my visits, but the quality of Betty's life was deteriorating. She was unable to manage the TV; the ViewClix which provided her with revolving pictures of friends and family also proved too complicated. She loved the AeroGarden, but she couldn't remember when or how much to water. And her Blackberry became too difficult to manage. She tended to wear the same clothes, bathed less frequently, and left half-eaten meals in the refrigerator. Her room didn't get cleaned as well or as often as I would have liked, and the flowers I brought her prematurely wilted in their vase for lack of attention. Although I was not living with Betty, the amount of attention I paid to her and the staff felt like a part time job.

Then COVID hit, right when she was experiencing an increased amount of sundowning. As mask requirements, vaccinations, and in-room quarantines settled around her, loneliness and depression worsened. Prevented from leaving her room for long periods, she struggled to get through the days, unable to comprehend what was happening. My visits ceased for months, but I was able to secure the services of a caregiver whom we had originally gotten to know as a server in the dining room. Danielle was a jolly person who exuded friendliness and compassion. Dr. Dan and I asked her if she would be interested in staying with Betty during the late afternoons and evening hours when Betty's moods tended to darken. CHAL allowed her to be hired by us on an hourly basis. I think she saved Betty's life. She wasn't a trained caregiver by any means, but her understanding of the human condition and her innate ability to sense and respond to Betty's AD-induced behaviors made her the perfect person. She cajoled Betty to get outside and walk and persuaded her to recount her experiences as teacher and traveler. She established a level of trust, frequently reminding Betty that she was loved even though her son and I were unable to visit. Because she was considered an essential worker, Danielle was allowed to enter CHAL while the pandemic raged.

Danielle provided Dr. Dan and me with weekly updates on Betty for the better part of a year. As COVID wreaked havoc on CHAL's resident population and staff, we were able to get a sense of how Betty was surviving. She never contracted the virus, but her overall mental condition took a hit, even with Danielle going out of her way to keep her spirits up. She began fantasizing about her sister who had died thirty years earlier, and she had difficulty staying up in winter months when the days were shorter. When staff removed her favorite chair from the main entrance, she was distraught. Her QMAP changed every other day, causing Betty to feel frightened when confronted by new personnel entering her room to dole out her medications, sometimes without knocking. Occasionally, she just locked her door.

Danielle did her best but under the COVID restrictions, she was fighting an uphill battle to keep Betty's spirits up. She continued to be creative, bringing sticker puzzle books to Betty, going over old picture albums, taking walks in the building when the weather was inclement and persuading Betty to take an occasional shower. She earned Betty's trust, but she was unwilling to abide by CHAL's demand that all caregivers be vaccinated. She was forced to terminate her work with Betty, and we found ourselves once again looking for experienced help. There were several companies in Denver which provided caregivers, and we gave a few of them a try. But after Danielle, no one seemed to match her knowledge of AD, her innate sensitivity, or the desire to learn. We were back to babysitters.

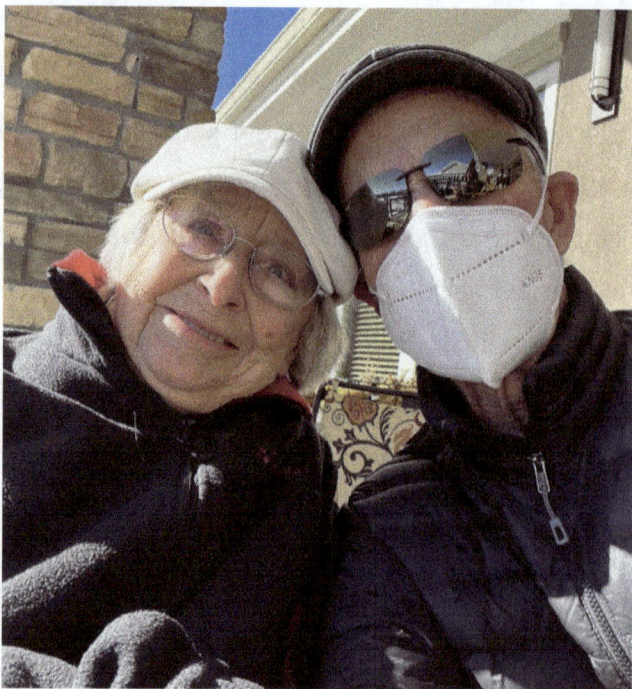

*Back to CHAL during COVID*

By the winter of 2021–2022, I was able to return to CHAL, and what I encountered was devastating. Betty was glad to have me back in her life even with a mask on. She was physically weak and mentally run-down, but she was delighted to resume ice cream outings, a few short walks, and hand-holding on the porch. It became clear to me that her condition was not good enough to remain in assisted living much longer. In fact, CHAL's director hinted that she would have to be removed to memory care if she stayed in the facility. I did not want to move her to memory care, because CHAL had neither the staff nor sufficient medical personnel on board to properly manage its memory care department. At least that was my opinion. We needed another solution.

Fortunately, Dr. Dan had decided to retire. In the spring of 2022, he came for a visit and concluded that it was time to take Mom home to Hawaii. I was totally surprised when he announced his intention. I felt a mixture of relief and sadness. When he and Patty returned a few months later to clean out Betty's apartment in preparation for the flight to Hawaii, I made one last trip to CHAL to say goodbye. It was a wrenching moment. Betty didn't know that it was our final goodbye, but I held her fiercely and wept like a baby. She was going home, but she would be in my heart forever. Perhaps that sounds melodramatic, but I have learned from others that because "the long goodbye" is long and infused with so many attempts to ease the suffering caused by a damnable disease, the emotional power of goodbyes can be overwhelming. I knew that it would be terribly hard on both of us were I to maintain a relationship with Betty when she left for Hawaii. The goodbye at CHAL was, indeed, final.

Everyone was concerned about the actual move. Betty was not in the best of health to travel. She had experienced an emotional collapse prior to Dr. Dan's arrival and had to be hospitalized for a few days. Even with Dr. Dan and Patty overseeing the move, I was afraid that in Betty's weakened condition, the trip might be too much for her.

But she did fine. It was Dr. Dan who had the problems. When their plane landed in Hawaii, Dr. Dan tested positive for COVID and immediately quarantined himself in his own home. The next day, Patty took Betty to the CCRC at which they had made a reservation. Because she had been close to Dr. Dan during

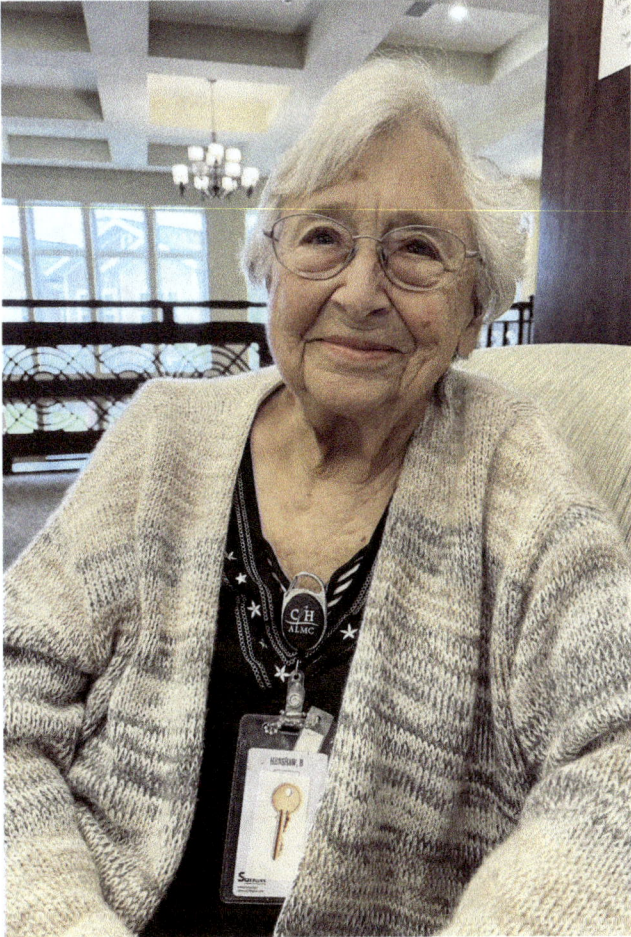

*Betty just prior to leaving for Hawaii*

the recent flight, Betty was quarantined in her room under lock and key. She was terrified and ended up banging on the door all night long.

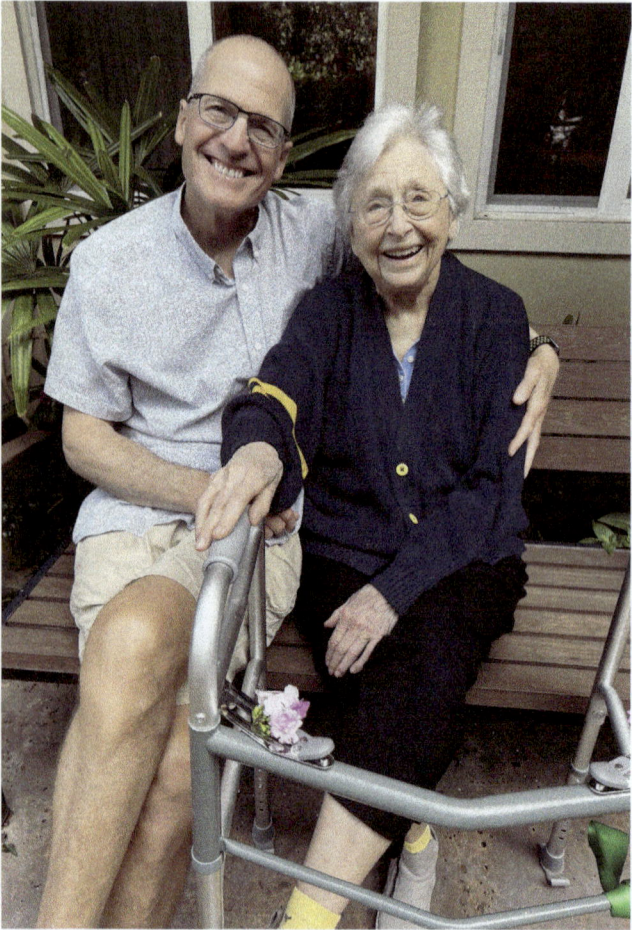

*Betty with Dr. Dan*

The next day, she was sent back to Dr. Dan where she remained for six weeks until another facility announced an opening. During that time,

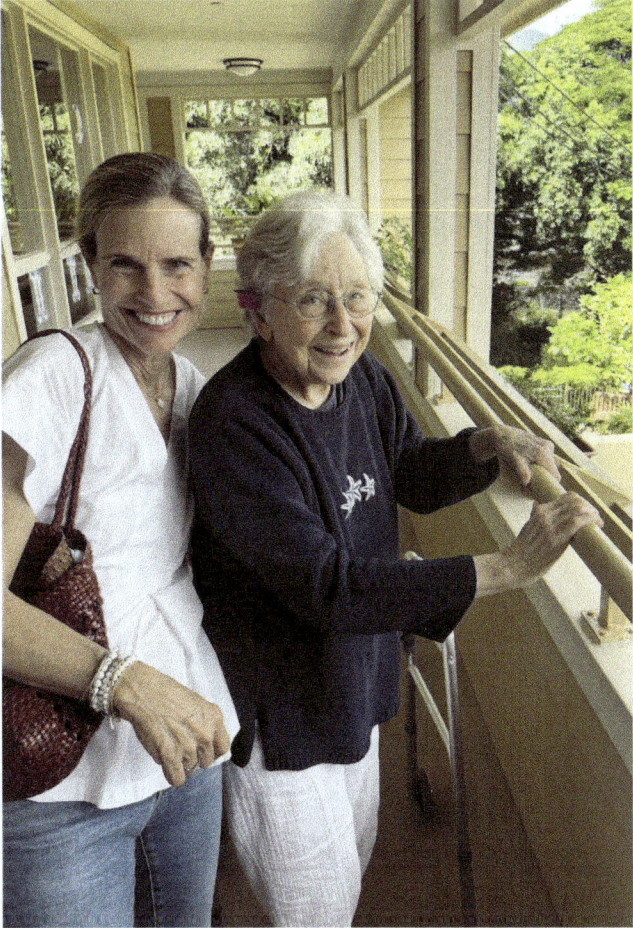

*Betty with Patty at Hale Ku'ike*

Dr. Dan came down with an attack of shingles, Patty fell and broke a bone in her wrist, and Betty repeatedly declared she was bored and asked where all the people were. Hale Ku'ike in nearby Kaneohe offered space just in time. The small memory care facility for 12 residents turned out to have both the environment and the personnel suitable for Betty's condition. There were multiple colorful gardens, a nice porch for Betty to enjoy the outdoors, and dedicated staff who had worked there for extended periods. Betty settled in quickly and with frequent visits from her son and daughter-in-law, she adapted to her new home with relative ease.

CCRCs everywhere deal with the employee turnover issue, but in Hawaii that problem is less dramatic, because the elderly (kūkū or kupuna ) are traditionally respected and treated with love by younger generations. This powerful cultural tradition has the result of providing caregivers with an intuitive head start on how to treat older people with dementia. Most Hawaiians can't afford the $75,000 a year required to place a loved one with AD in a memory care facility, but because of the examples set in their own families, they are better prepared to serve as caregivers in facilities for those with dementia and other age-related conditions.

They know that people with dementia can live a long time. As I write this in the spring of 2024, Betty has been living with AD for a dozen years and has turned 88. She has been in two very different facilities for 6 of those 12 years, and her family has been willing to pay the extraordinary cost of her care, which has been mercurial at best. But for most people who lack the resources to provide this level of care, the only alternative is for family members to assume responsibility along with the stress of internal family frictions, petty jealousies, and a lack of agreement on how best to deal with the irrational and unpredictable behaviors associated with dementia. The responsibility of caregiving can result in disastrous consequences for all concerned: emotional, physical, social, financial.

But the rise of reported cases of dementia worldwide suggests that more and more Baby Boomers, Gen X, Millennials, and Gen Z are likely to face this challenge at some point in their lives. It would be nice if they were able to count on professional assistance with the caregiving requirements they will face. As of 2023, about 11% of Americans over 65 have AD. More than 1,300 Americans develop this condition daily. That's one person every 65 seconds. Worldwide, it is estimated that the number of people with dementia will double every 20 years, reaching 150,000,000 people by 2050. According to Alzheimer's Disease International, 10 million new cases of AD are diagnosed worldwide every year, while three quarters of the people who have AD are never diagnosed. In the United States, the recognized number of AD sufferers is in the range of 7 million, with the West and Southeast expected to incur the largest increase. Almost two thirds of Americans diagnosed with dementia are women; Blacks and Hispanics remain statistically more vulnerable.

So, what's causing this explosion? Experts can't agree. Some say it's due to our living longer; others blame changing climate, lifestyles, genetics, and air pollution. Yet the 2023 Alzheimer's Association Report notes that there are ". . . currently no FDA approved treatments that prevent or cure Alzheimer's disease. . . ." The scientific research community has noted the important role of amyloid proteins in the development of dementia but as of this writing, there are no drugs that can postpone or prevent dementia from running its murderous course. The bottom line is that there is no cure for AD and there is no agreement on the cause of AD.

The Alzheimer's Association does good work, and it raises a lot of money. But based on my personal experience and what I know about the current state of AD research, the Association should spend more time and use more of its assets to develop professional caregivers. Most families will try to keep their loved ones at home but to succeed, they need assistance from people who understand the idiosyncracies of this condition and how best to make patients more content and comfortable as it progresses. At present, the Association's appeal letters focus on the need for donations to achieve a cure. Obviously, research must continue and a cure must be the goal. But until the true cause is identified and agreed upon, FDA-approved drugs will provide only temporary, marginal relief at best. By contrast, a well-trained caregiver (family member or hired professional) can provide an AD sufferer with enormous amounts of comfort and reassurance far beyond the power of current drugs.

In her 2019 book *Dementia with Dignity*, Judy Cornish makes a powerful argument for keeping AD patients at home as long as possible. In the United States, 22 million families may be exposed to some form of dementia by 2030, she notes; 40 million by 2040. "We can't afford to carry on the way we have been, believing that warehousing people in long-term care facilities and quieting their distress with psychotropic drugs is appropriate." Because dementia is the most likely health issue families will face in coming decades—and also the most expensive, more likely and more costly, in fact, than cancer or heart disease—common sense demands a radically different approach. With Medicare unwilling to help unless nursing is involved and Medicaid out of the picture until a family's resources are exhausted, it's time to develop a different strategy: professionally trained caregivers who can assist families in their homes.

A community college program to certify caregivers would focus on the emotional component of dementia. The medical community has tended to see AD as an anxiety-related disease. There is no doubt that anxiety is a very common behavior, but caregivers who have the proper psychological training can use their skills to decrease the frequency of anxiety by concentrating more on sensory and social stimulation. They can be trained to understand the intuitive part of the brain: senses, hunches, gut feelings, instincts, etc. They can comprehend the role of abstract reasoning and how it relates to creativity, instantaneous thinking, recognition of beauty, and intuition. They can understand why the past and the future are of less importance than the present, and they can develop the skills necessary to develop trust with someone who has become angry and suspicious. Caregiving can be directed at supporting emotional needs, obviating the old approach of trying to restore or treat the absence of linear thought and behavior.

The goal of caregiving should be dignity. You would think that every caregiver would understand that, but lots of things get in the way: impatience, a desire to restore aspects of an old relationship, asking too many questions, trying to restore common sense and logic in the brain of an AD sufferer, being in a bad mood, etc. To simplify their work, caregivers sometimes tend to treat dementia sufferers as irresponsible adolescents prone to abnormal and irresponsible behavior. Of course, there is always the possibility for erratic conduct, but the more secure they feel and the less they are judged, the better the chance that they will respond with less drama.

In my experience, Betty was treated both

at home and in the CCRCs with considerable respect. Some of the most devoted caregivers in her life gave much of themselves and provided Betty with the dignity she deserved. But all too often, these same people had to leave the business. They became too emotionally involved and found it difficult to separate the affection they felt from the job they were hired to do. This is certainly understandable, but I would contend that if a professional caregiving program were established, those with the right amount of empathy would see it through and would be able to deal with the emotional stresses of the job when hired. Others who drop by the wayside would do so in recognition of their vulnerabilities.

I want to close by saying that this love story has a happy ending. After two years in Hawaii, it is clear that Betty is well and well cared for. She is close to her son, she is a resident in a small and professionally run community, her health is reasonably good, and she is surrounded by a natural environment that brings her peace.

Looking back over our ten years living with Alzheimer's, I am able to reflect on how much I learned about the human condition and about myself. I grieve often for the loss I feel, but I am a little wiser about happily-ever-after endings. By arguing for a more professional cadre of caregivers, I hope to make clear both the inevitable increase in AD and the unrealistic concept of CCRCs which all too frequently can drain family assets. I am fully aware that professionally trained caregivers will mean a higher cost for homecare. But that expense will be a fraction of what the CCRCs charge, and there is every expectation that someone with AD can achieve a higher level of contentment in familiar surroundings than in a for-profit institution. I am sad that AD destroyed the incredibly beautiful relationship Betty and I experienced. But how could I ever be anything but grateful for the love and gentleness she brought to my life? The mark on my soul is indelible. In some way, I know that we will meet again.

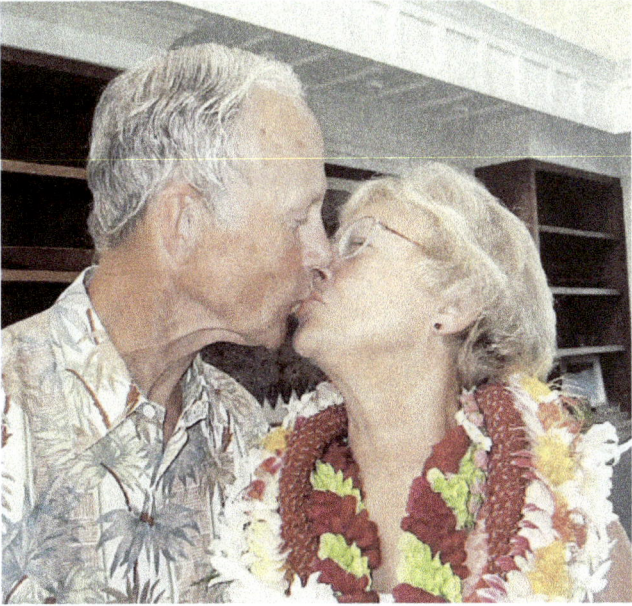

*The kiss*

# SELECT RESOURCES

The following is a list of references with which I am personally familiar and from which I have benefited over the course of my experience as a caregiver.

## BOOKS

Cornish, Judy. *Dementia With Dignity. Living Well with Alzheimer's or Dementia.* Scott's Valley, CA: Create Space Independent Publishing Platform, 2019.

> A guidebook that provides information on how to keep people at home as they evolve through stages of dementia. Check out Cornish's website which has a great deal of related information.

Doraiswamy, P. Murali, Lisa P. Gwyther and Tina Adler. *The Alzheimer Action Plan. What You Need to Know—And What You Can Do—About Memory Problems From Prevention to Early*

*Intervention and Cure.* New York: St. Martin's Griffin, 2009.

This is a powerful book on how to know if someone has dementia, what the best treatments are, and how to cope when faced with the responsibility of caregiving.

Genova, Lisa. *Still Alice.* New York: Simon & Schuster, Inc. 2007.

A work of fiction, this is a powerful story about a Columbia professor who describes the gradual loss of her ability to communicate and her feelings of disorientation as dementia becomes increasingly severe. The author's ability to articulate the suffering of the professor's caregiving children who watch the process unfold makes this novel uncannily real and worthy of being read by all.

Koenig Coste, Joanne. *Learning to Speak Alzheimer's.* New York: Houghton Mifflin Harcourt Publishing Co., 2003.

This is a practical approach to enhancing the

wellbeing of both dementia sufferers and caregivers. The author stresses the importance of a caregiver's need to communicate with patients in their own reality with the objective of improving two-way discourse.

Mace, Nancy L. and Peter V. Rabbins. *The 36-Hour Day*. New York City: Grand Central Life and Style, 2012.

A great book for families who are caring for people with dementia. It focuses on the importance of acceptance, instead of attempting behavioral change, and urges caregivers to have a sense of humor.

Miles, Margaret R. *The Long Goodbye. Dementia Diaries*. Atlanta: Cascade Books, 2017.

The author describes a creative approach to loving dementia patients. She argues that it is possible to "make" rather than just endure a dementia patient's daily existence, while at the same time having new and valuable life experiences.

Power, Allen. *Dementia Beyond Drugs.* Baltimore: Health Professions Press, 2010.

Reducing the use of psychotropic drugs is the focus of this work. The author believes that medications are not the way to lessen stress experienced by individuals living with dementia. Instead, he presents ways that caregivers can accomplish much more than drugs, producing outcomes that are more beneficial for everyone.

## OTHER SOURCES

https://www.alz.org

This is a general website for anyone with questions about dementia. Experts can be contacted via a helpline (800-272-3900). They can answer just about any question with cogent advice and they are able to provide beginning caregivers with in-home guidelines. They are also able to direct caregivers to local Alzheimer's Association chapters.

https://www.alzheimers.gov

> More specifically aimed at caregivers, this website reviews publications, directions for improving care of a family member, and tips from the CDC and NIH as to how home care can be improved.

https://www.adear@nia.nih.gov

> ADEAR (Alzheimer's and Related Dementias Education and Referral Center) is a service of the National Institute on Aging and the National Institute of Health. It provides assistance to caregivers.

https://www.aarp.org

> This website is filled with suggestions on how to manage the behaviors of dementia sufferers. It also describes the benefits of therapeutic fibbing in order for caregivers to be able to meet their patients in their own reality.

https://www.cdc.gov/aging/publications/features/
alzheimers_caregivers.html

In this website there are references to
programs that can improve caregiver skills,
especially in the area of communications
and in creative ways to resolve problems.

## ABOUT THE AUTHOR

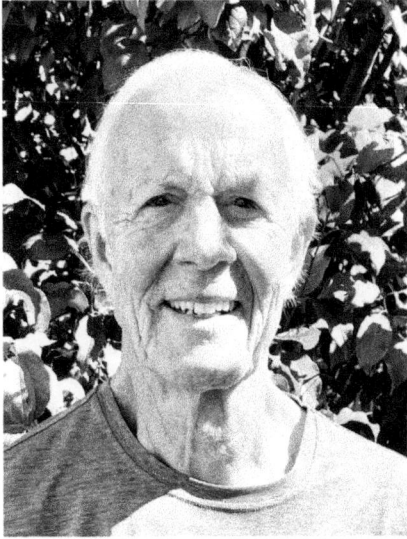

Daniel Tyler is a retired history professor. Born before WWII, he grew up on a ranch in Colorado prior to studying at Harvard College. After receiving a degree in political science and a commission in the USAF, he served as a jet flight instructor and taught history in Hawaii. Tyler returned to ranching for a few years then earned a Ph.D. in American History. He taught in Mexico, Argentina, and at Colorado State University where he researched the West's water development and resulting conflict. Previous publications by Daniel Tyler include, *The Last Water Hole in the West*, *WD Farr, Cowboy in the Boardroom*, *Silver Fox of the Rockies*, *Love in an Envelope*, *Bucks County's Benevolent Squire*, and *Looking Back At Ninety*.

www.ingramcontent.com/pod-product-compliance
Lightning Source LLC
La Vergne TN
LVHW022341080426
835508LV00012BA/1301

9 781963 117103